The Adventures of Sugar The Travelling Bear.

Written by Donna-Michelle Hall.

Illustrated by Alena Mae Donkin.

ISBN:1984188925
ISBN-13:9781984188922

DEDICATION.

Well, the story you are about to read is actually kind of true, because there is indeed a real life cuddly teddy bear called Sugar, who does indeed travel round the world and he visits children for a little while to share their fun and adventures. He visits very special children, like you, who have type one diabetes. Of course, this is why my girls and I named him Sugar, because as you are about to learn, or may already know, type one diabetes means your body cannot control the amount of sugar in your blood without help.

Sugar is a very treasured bear, who lets children know that they too are very special, and he knows that they need to be brave a lot of the time, so Sugar is on hand to give lots of bear hugs and to help the children, and you, feel less alone.

Sugar is actually one of fifty bears that I have sent all over the world to visit children with type one diabetes. The bears are having adventures across the UK, Northern Ireland, America, Australia, Africa, Iceland, Portugal, France, Canada and beyond since my own daughter developed type one diabetes. The bears all share adventures with the families that they stay with, and they help children with type one diabetes feel less alone, and to feel like part of a community of people who all share the same condition.

***Parents/Carers please find extra support on my Facebook page 'The Insulin Gang' or to get your child involved in having a bear, 'The Adventures of the Insulin Gang Travelling Bears' also on Facebook. Both closed groups for privacy.*

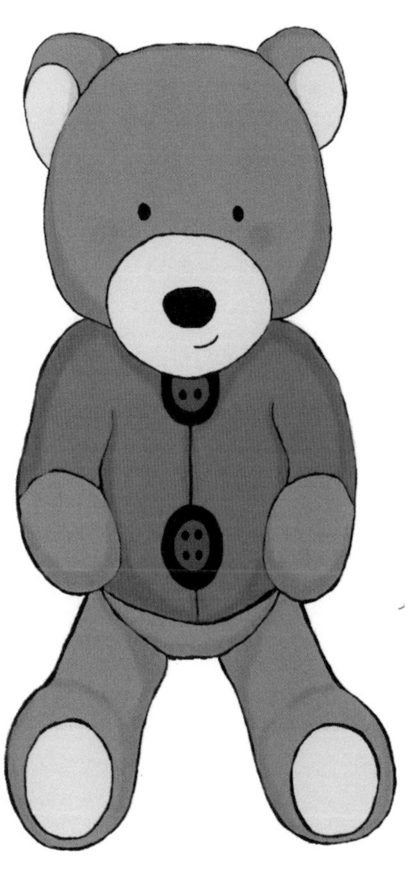

CONTENTS.

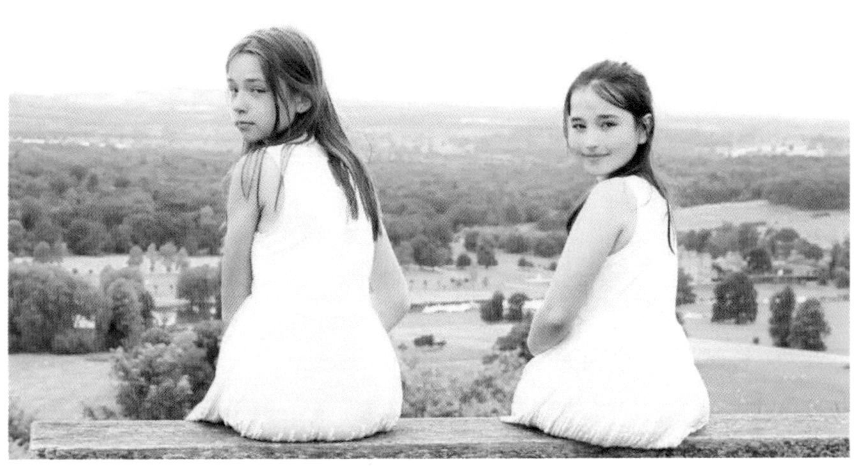

Cerys is on the left, and Alena on the right. Cerys is my reason for the development of the Insulin Gang support group and the Travelling Bears. Alena is her biggest supporter.

ACKNOWLEDGMENTS

I feel it only appropriate to acknowledge my beautiful daughter Cerys-Anne who this book is based on. Cerys was diagnosed with type one diabetes aged 9 years old, and some 7 years later she astounds me with her attitude to life, learning and to others, she really is quite a remarkable person, of whom I am deeply proud. Cerys is a high achiever and is probably one of the most compassionate people I know. She will go very far in life.

I would also like to acknowledge my other daughter Alena Mae who provided me with the illustrations for this book. Alena herself has a health issue to contend with, and has for the last few years lived with M.E. Life is challenging for her and school is not possible right now, but Alena amazes me with her sheer grit and determination and her desire to keep on learning, applying herself and making a difference to others. Alena is such a talented Artist, and I am so proud of her maturity, fairness and attitude shown to others. I am deeply proud that despite their own health challenges the girls both aim high and achieve.

I also must acknowledge the type one community and the members of my support groups, The Insulin Gang, and The Adventures of the Insulin Gang Travelling Bears, where there is such a strong sense of community and togetherness, where we all really root for each other, in a place where we provide friendship, education and a sense of morale. I think the type one community is a force to be reckoned with and we are proud to be a part of it.

SUGAR XX

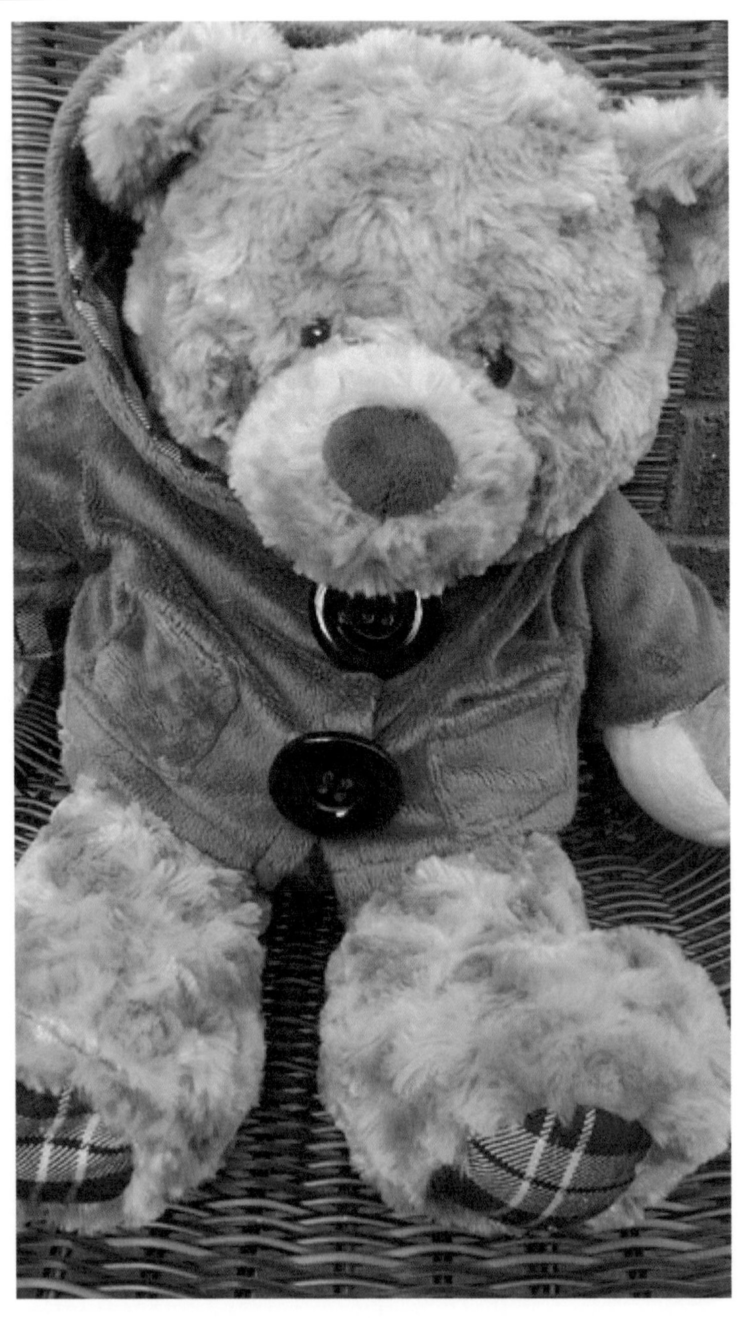

1. SUGAR THE BEAR GOES TO HOSPITAL.

Sugar the bear lives with Anna, a nurse. Anna is a children's nurse. Sugar often stays with Anna. Sugar is a very friendly looking bear. He is always very smart looking, his fur is always well brushed and soft, and his velvet green jacket buttoned.

He prides himself on being a well dressed bear and he takes his role very seriously.

His role is to help children.

Sugar the bear is going on a very important journey today. He is going to go and visit a child who is staying in a hospital near to where he lives.

Sugar sits patiently waiting for Anna the nurse to collect him from the kitchen chair and to take him to the children's hospital. Anna has been a nurse for a very long time. She is very friendly and good at her job.

Sugar knows that the hospital is a place where poorly children can be made to feel much better. He also knows that hospitals can make some children feel worried, so he has a very special job today. He is looking forward to visiting a little girl called Cerys-Anne. She went into the hospital just yesterday and is understandably feeling a bit scared.

Cerys-Anne is nine years old and is feeling a bit fed up. Anna knows that a visit from Sugar will help to cheer Cerys-Anne up. Anna picks Sugar up from her kitchen chair, brushes his fur quickly, gives him a wink, and heads off to the hospital.

Cerys-Anne has been very poorly for a long time with a chest infection, and after visiting her doctor she has been brought in to the hospital, because the doctor discovered she has sugar in her blood. This means she needs to have some extra tests.

Cerys and her parents are a bit worried, but they know that Cerys is in safe hands.

The doctors in the hospital tells Cerys-Anne that she has got type one diabetes, and this makes Cerys feel worried. The doctors gently explain that inside her body there is a something called a pancreas, and normally this organ makes very special hormones including insulin. Something has made Cerys' pancreas stop making insulin, the doctors think it was the chest infection, and the pancreas will not start making insulin again.

This news makes Cerys and her parents feel quite surprised and sad. They feel shocked and Mum wonders whether she had done something wrong at all. Dad said he felt worried. They did not realise that children could develop type one diabetes and did not know any other children with it. They wondered how they would manage and Mum felt tearful. So did Cerys. All of these feelings are very normal.

The doctors and nurses will help Cerys and her parents to understand all of these feelings and worries, and to realise that this has not happened because of anything anyone did. No one made this happen. This is not to do with too little exercise or too much sugary food, not at all. No one could have made this happen to Cerys, and no one could have stopped it. In this case, the chest infection Cerys had been suffering with caused her body to damage her pancreas.

The doctors and nurses will talk to Cerys-Anne and her parents and help them learn how to manage type one diabetes by themselves once they get home. Other people that look after Cerys-Anne will need to be taught these things too.

There is a lot to learn and a lot to remember, but it is okay, nurses will keep in touch from now on and will help them to remember and things will all start to make sense soon.

Cerys though is feeling poorly and tired, and sits on the hospital bed and begins to cry. She is not sure what is happening to her and wishes she had brought her favourite bear because she always holds him when she is sad.

Anna arrives just in time and introduces herself then quickly passes Sugar the bear to Cerys-Anne to hold. Anna gives Cerys a kind smile and says everything will be okay.

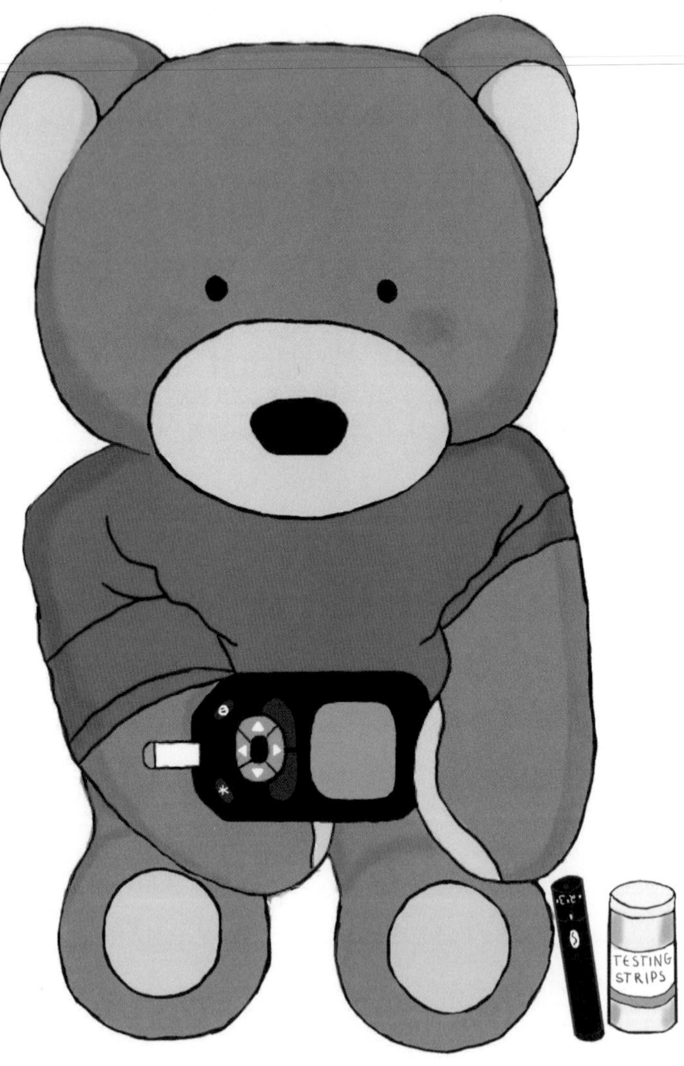
TESTING
STRIPS

Anna puts a little hospital bracelet on Sugar and writes his name on it, just like the one Cerys-Anne has, to keep him safe. Cerys has always loved bears but, in their rush to get to hospital, all hers were left on her bed at home. She pressed her face into Sugars and tears fell fast. Sugar knew she was sad and so hugged her back, with a lot of love, and wanted her to know she was going to be alright. Cerys squeezed Sugar so tightly, and she did not want to let him go.

Anna the nurse gently talked to Cerys and her parents about how they would need to test her blood sugar levels regularly with a very clever little machine, and that they would need to prick her finger to make it bleed a little, and Cerys will need injections of insulin every day. Cerys is scared of needles but the nurse shows her how tiny the needles are, and Cerys feels less afraid, especially as her Mummy and Daddy both have a turn at testing their blood.

The Adventures of Sugar, the Travelling Bear.

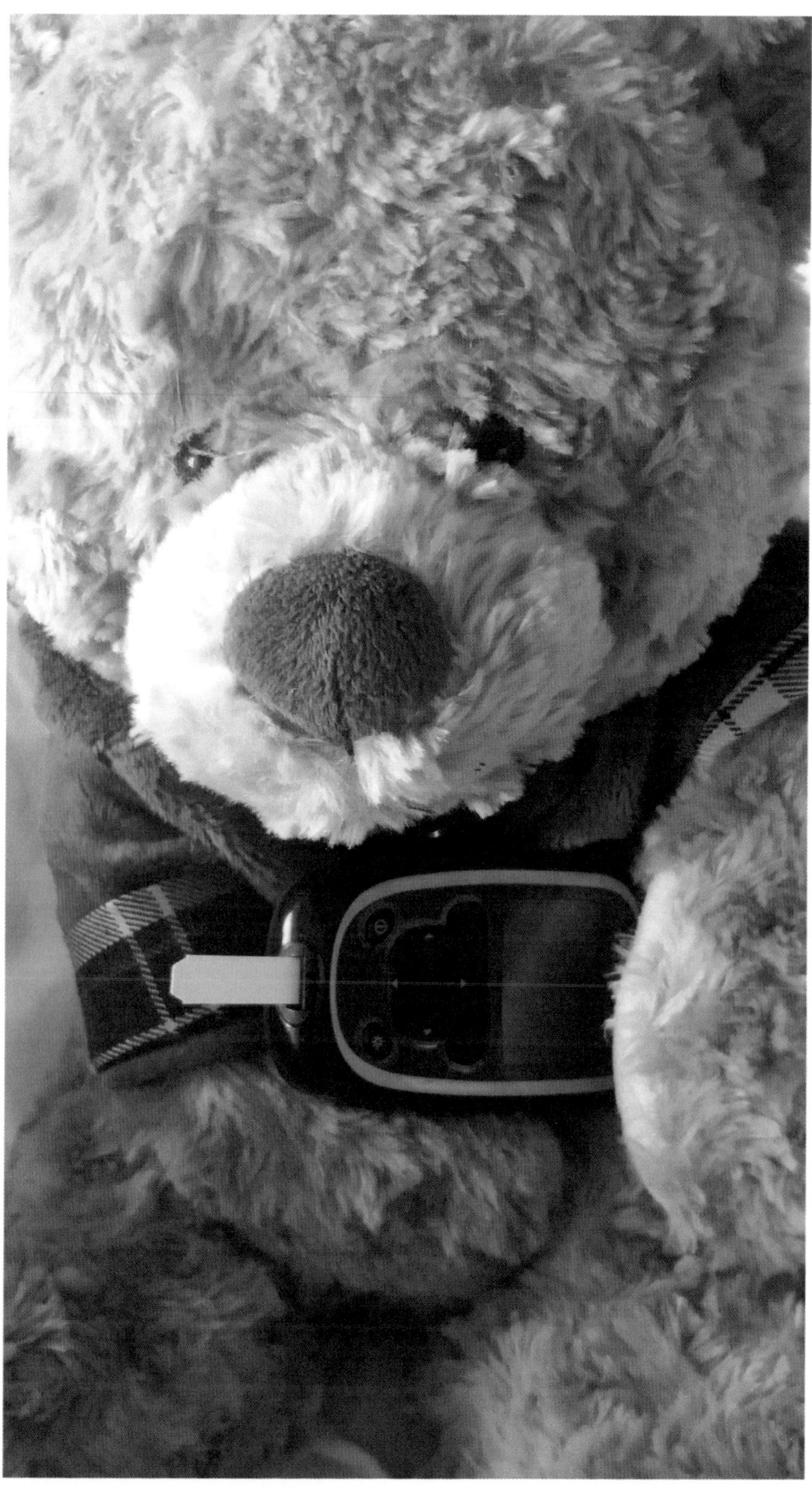

Sugar the bear has visited lots of children with type one diabetes. Sometimes he gets taken into hospital so often that he feels quite tired. He does know that there are other bears like him, all over the world, who visit children and help them to manage their diabetes. Even though children like Cerys have left hospital, they can still feel scared at times, or need to be extra brave. There are lots of things to think about, and children have to have help from their teachers, families and friends at times. The Travelling Bears, are all very important, and their job is simple, to send smiles across the miles. To make children feel less alone. It is a job that they take very seriously indeed, and they all have a special bear telephone which they call each other on, whenever they can and they talk about the wonderful children that they meet with type one diabetes, and how the children make everyone so proud. Tommy, Connor, Joy, Carbo, Ryan, Duffy, Gluco, Teddy Ryder, Frederick, Dex and Pumpi are just some of the other bears that are travelling the world.

The bears all help children who feel lonely, or worried, and the bears even get taken to hospital appointments and school. They are always very smartly dressed for their adventures.

The bears, although very different from each-other, and visiting very different parts of the world, all have one very special secret that no adults know, apart from Anna the nurse. The bears all have the same special secret. At night, they come alive and have special adventures when most other people are sleeping.

Sugar can talk to the children if they happen to be awake but every morning he scatters special sparkly magic dust on to them, and they forget that he is actually a talking, walking bear. This means Sugar can be even more helpful, and has many great adventures.

Sugar knows that even though Cerys is feeling sad at the moment, he will help to remind her to smile.

Anna carefully explained to Cerys that from now on when Cerys eats she would need Mummy or Daddy to work out how much insulin she would need for each meal or snack. The insulin would have to be given to Cerys in an injection. The needle on the injection is very small. Cerys did not like needles. Anna helped her and her Mum and Dad practice putting the needles into an orange.

The Adventures of Sugar, the Travelling Bear.

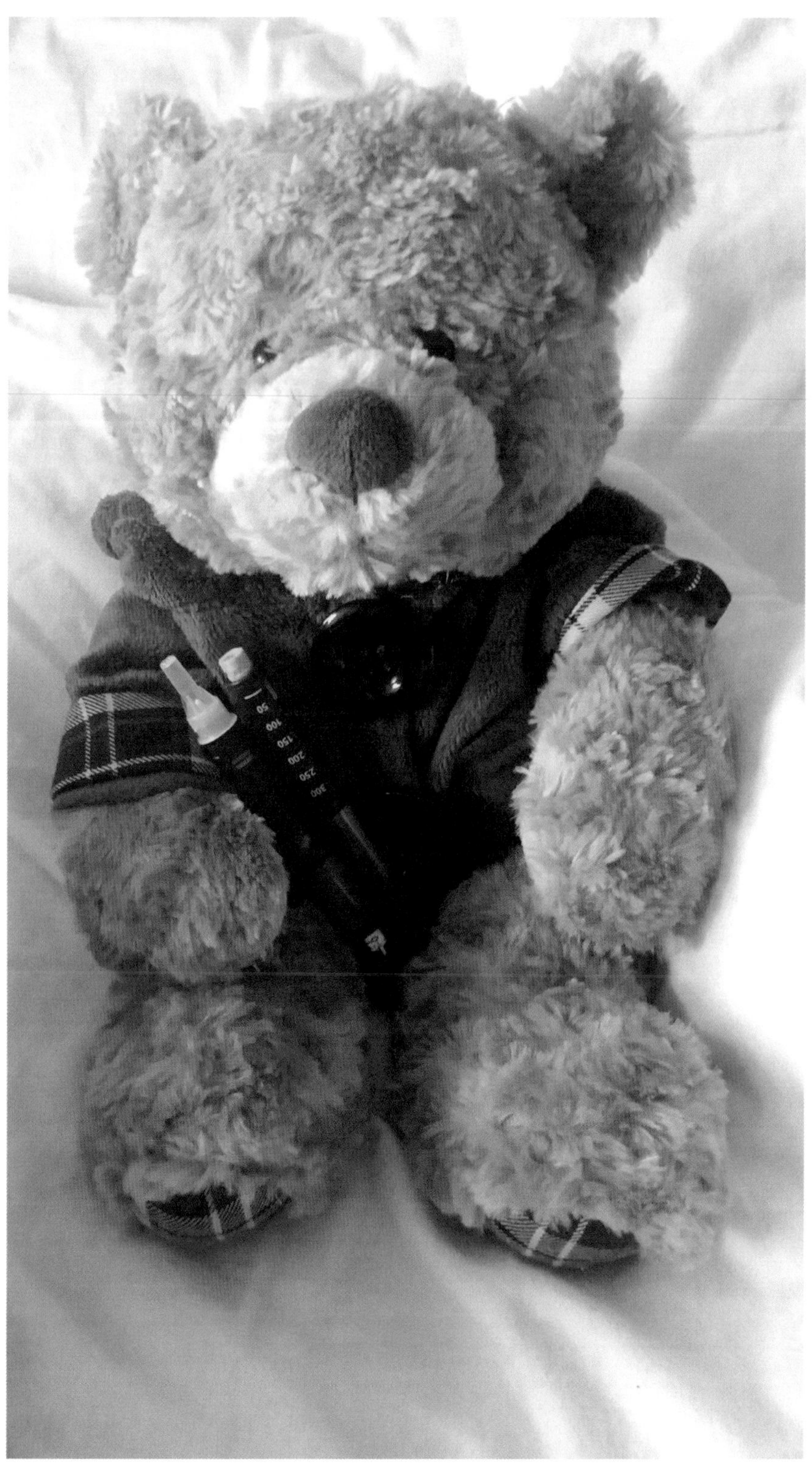

They spent a long time doing this until they felt better about how to do it properly. As Cerys gets older she will be able to do this herself. Cerys thought this sounded quite worrying and like hard work, and Mummy thought she would need to be extra careful with maths when working out what insulin was needed. It had to be done very carefully Anna explained, as too much or too little insulin could make Cerys feel poorly.

Everyone feels tired. It has been a long day with lots to learn, so Mummy and Daddy decide to go home to catch up on some sleep. Mummy and Daddy said goodbye to Cerys after lots of hugs and kisses.

Cerys does not want them to leave really but knows that she is in the care of some lovely nurses and she leapt back on to her bed holding on tightly to Sugar the Bear.

Sugar almost seemed to hug Cerys-Anne tightly back as she snuggled down into her bed, tired from a very busy day. Her eyes grew heavy and she soon fell fast asleep.

This is of course when Sugar decided to work some magic. He wriggled gently from Cerys' hands and sat on the edge of the bed. He knew that she was worried about everything she had heard today and he understood why. He wanted to help her though.

Sugar knew of a special book that would help Cerys and her parents learn about different foods and how they could work out how much insulin each food would need. Lots of foods have something inside called 'car bo hy drate'. (carbohydrate) It's a big word and it's very important but Cerys will learn it quickly enough

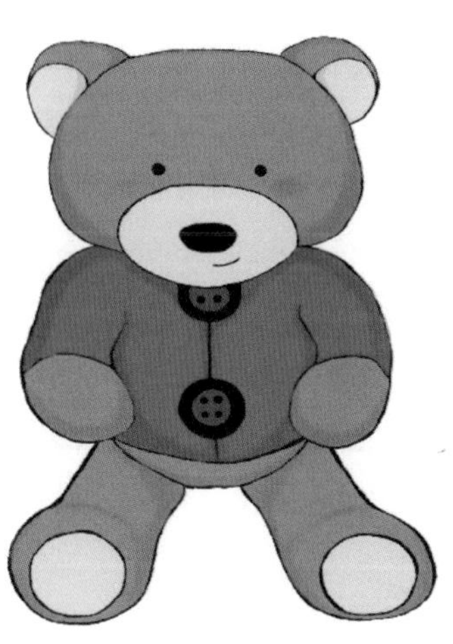

In the special book that Sugar reaches from a shelf it has pictures of all different foods.

It is heavy and Sugar pulls it along the floor to take it to the bed, and he has to stretch up high and climb hard to get himself and the book back on the bed. He knows that Cerys will be shocked when he wakes her, but he tugs at her pyjama sleeve until she opens her eyes. She stares at him, and thinks that she is dreaming.

Cerys rubs her eyes in disbelief. She blinks hard and Sugar says, "Hello Cerys, do not be alarmed, I wake up every night when most of the adults are sleeping or busy working. I am here to help you," Sugar smiles warmly at a sleepy Cerys and says, "Thank you for letting me help you lately and hug you."

Cerys still thinks she must be dreaming but she sees that Sugar is holding a heavy book so she helps him lift it properly onto the bed. Sugar says, "This book will help you learn about sugar and how eating different foods will affect the sugar in your blood." He holds the book up and there are brightly coloured pictures of foods, and he and Cerys look through, and Cerys sees lots of numbers next to the food. None of it makes sense, and she is tired, but Sugar is humming softly and she feels sleepy but happy, and is excited now that Sugar is awake and talking.

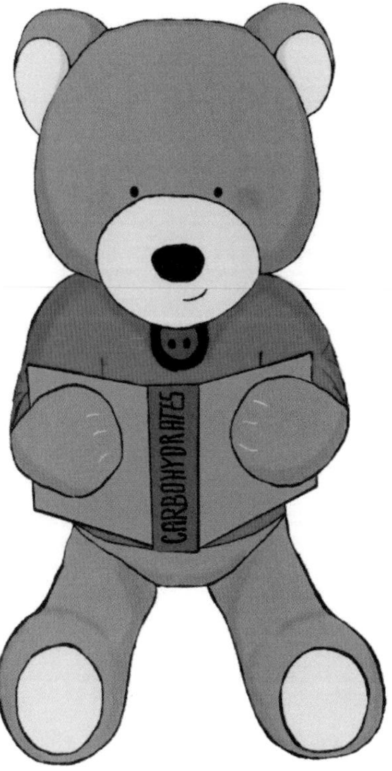
CARBOHYDRATES

Cerys and Sugar spend some time looking at the book and learning, and Sugar tells Cerys about all the other children he has met who have type one diabetes.

Sugar tells Cerys of children he knows who play football, ride horses, go on school holidays, visit diabetes camps, go to dance class, go swimming, travel. They all manage to do the things they used to be able to do, but things just take a little more planning now they have to manage diabetes.

Sugar tells Cerys lots of stories about other people he has met, children and adults, all who have type one diabetes.

Sugar once stayed with a man called Pete, who climbed to the top of a mountain recently, and also a lady called Louise who took Sugar all round America on the back of her motorbike. Both grown-ups have type one diabetes, but still have lots of fun and happy times, they just need to look after themselves carefully to keep well.

Cerys loved Sugars sparkly eyes and kind face. He had lovely soft fur and he made her feel like everything would be okay. Cerys soon grew tired, and led down on the bed. Sugar knew Cerys needed to sleep and so he snuggled down with her and she held him tightly until the morning came. Sugar waited until sunrise and reached up his paw and blew the magic sparkly dust into Cerys' face to stop her remembering their chat and the fact that the night time had seen him come alive.

Sugar led back down and waited for the hustle and bustle of morning.

Cerys woke and had a strange feeling, a nice one, one with less worry, and she waited for her Mum and Dad to arrive.

The nurse came and explained that there would be a meeting today about food and insulin. Cerys felt less worried and strangely felt like she already knew something about this. She saw a big book hanging off the shelf and felt like she had seen it before.

Cerys-Anne looked at Sugar the bear who was sat on the chair and he almost seemed to smile at her. Cerys picked him up.

The nurse arrived and made Cerys' bed and grabbed the book muttering that they would need it. The nurse took Cerys' hand and they walked down the corridor to where Mummy and Daddy were waiting to meet them in a little side room.

There is a special man in the room called a Dietitian who knows all about food. He is called Bob. He is very friendly and talks about that big word 'carbohydrate' again. Bob takes the big book from the nurse and starts listing a few items of food and wonders if anyone else knows what carbohydrates are in each food.

To everyone's surprise Cerys seems to know a lot of answers and no one knows why, not even Cerys.

Of course, Sugar knows why and yes, he is smiling to himself and feeling very pleased, because he now knows for sure that although there is a lot to learn about diabetes, Cerys and her family are going to be just fine.

Cerys is pleased to learn she is allowed home soon, and Anna the nurse comes in to say goodbye.

Cerys' Mum has brought in two of her teddy bears from home, and Cerys hugs them tightly but not before she has said a huge goodbye to Sugar.

Cerys knows Sugar needs to go and help other children now, and although she feels sad to see him go she understands that other children need to meet him too. Cerys feels sure that Sugar is a very special little bear, and as Anna takes him from Cerys and winks at her, it seems perhaps Anna know that he is too.

Donna-Michelle Hall.

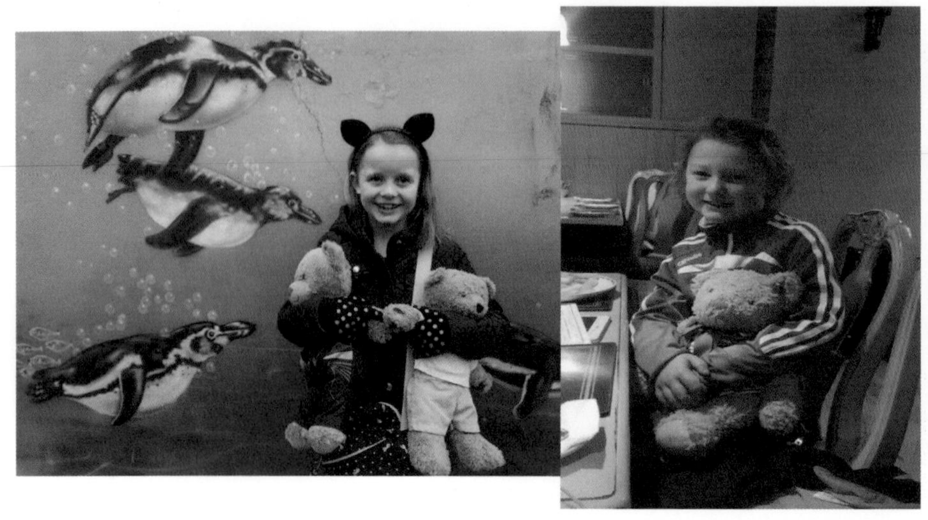

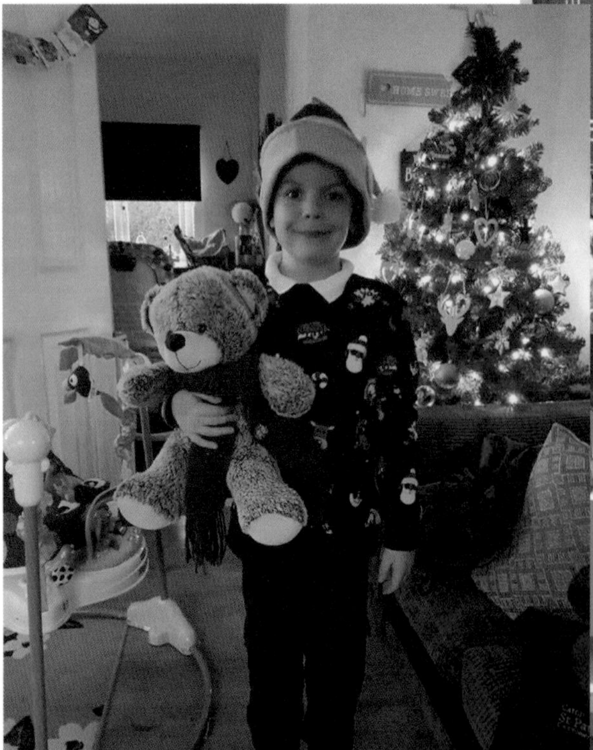

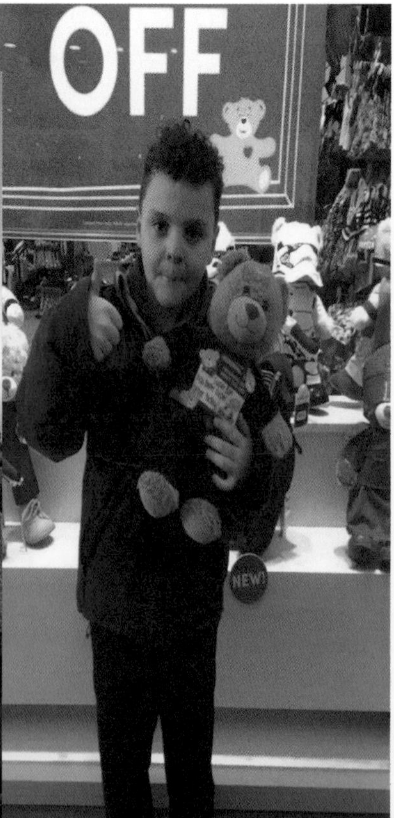

I really hope to share some more of Sugar's adventures with you again one day.

Remember, if you are reading this and you have type one diabetes, then look after yourself, and do not forget that type one diabetes or any other health issue does not define you. You have to respect it, and plan around it, but you are made up of so many wonderful qualities and type one diabetes is just a small part of you. You will go on to do amazing things, because I know, you are already amazing and life is full of exciting adventures for you.

Remember, if you are the parent, carer or friend to a child with type one diabetes, it is not always easy, and you are doing amazingly just by showing your support. The type one community is a force to be reckoned with, and you are part of that.

Take care, and have lots of fun.

From Donna, Cerys and Alena and all the travelling bears.

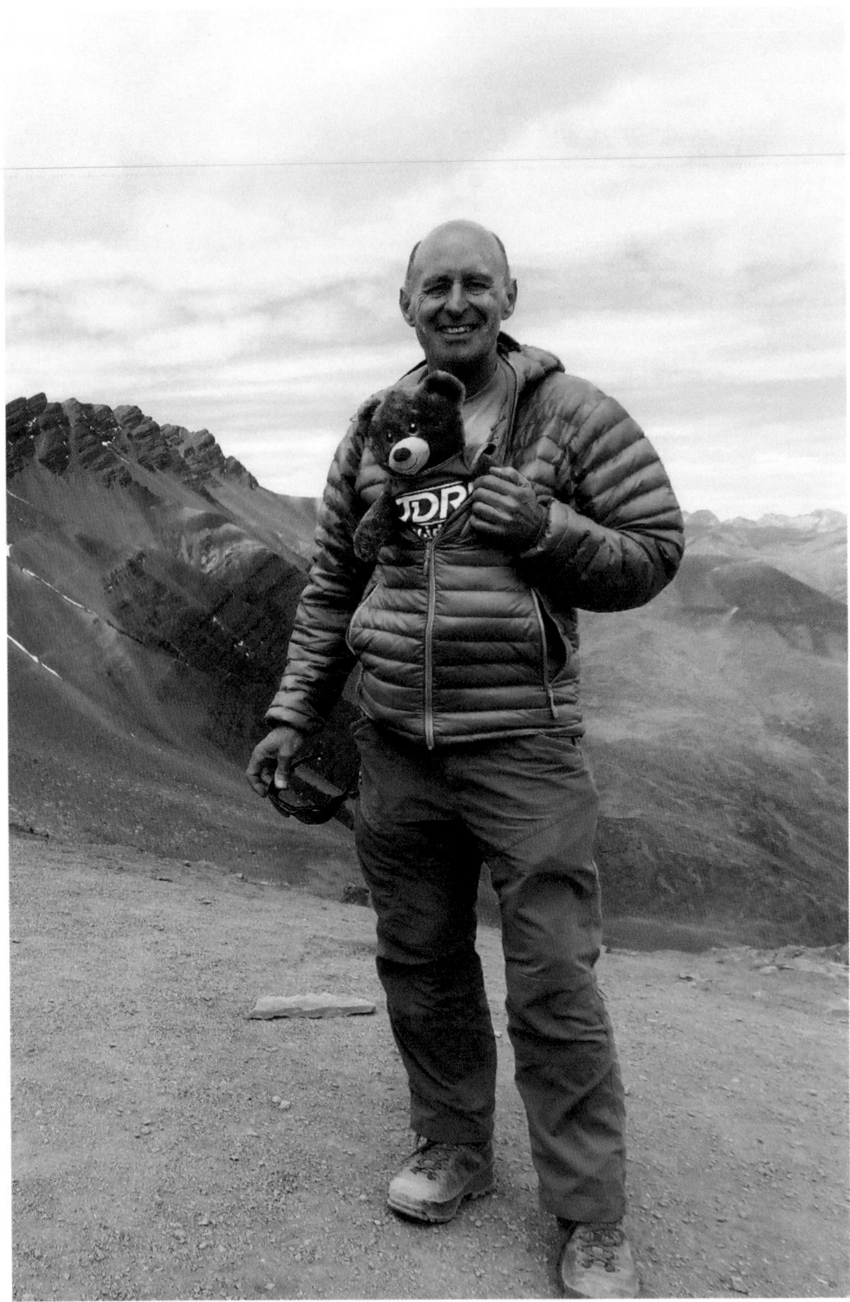

Pete climbed a mountain recently.

ABOUT THE AUTHOR.

I am mother to three children, all of whom make me incredibly proud with their achievements. Morgan my son is working towards becoming a Doctor, whilst Cerys is working towards becoming a Vet and Alena will brighten the world with her art for sure and wants to be a Teaching Assistant.

I feel incredibly lucky to have grown up in Wiltshire, and am in no real rush to ever leave it although if I do, it will be to escape to the coast! When my daughter Cerys was diagnosed with type one diabetes it was quite daunting for us. She was nine and needle phobic, it was not easy but with the support of some great people we have adapted and life with type one is our normal.

Since diagnosis brought feelings of needing to do something proactive to make a difference, as a family we began organising fundraising events and we have raised over ten thousand pounds mainly for diabetes charities. I also set up The Insulin Gang support group on Facebook and the Adventures of the Insulin Gang Travelling Bears which together with the fundraising events have brought some wonderful people into our life, too many to mention individually, but so many amazing people, many of whom we consider great friends.

I am at present studying for a Psychology and Counselling Degree with the Open University, it fits with my role at the moment as full time carer.

Family life is good, and our home is always filled with a lot of love and creativity.

I hope you enjoy this story and I hope other stories follow.

Printed in Great Britain
by Amazon